TABLE OF CONTENTS

PART ONE:
THE EFFECTIVE WAY TO GET HIRT

We have outlined 52 of our favourite exercises and why you should be doing them. You may not like or agree with them all but the purpose is to provide you with some basic physiological principles on why these exercises would be beneficial to you.

Before starting high intensity resistance training there are a few adjustments you need to make to exercise. In the past, you may have come to believe certain things about training, which may or may not be true.

These HIRT rules will put things into perspective from a physiological standpoint and clear up some of the myths that have become gospel in the fitness industry.

Let us now review the 10 basic HIRT principles to give you a grounding of high intensity resistance training.

01. Eliminate Unnecessary Exercises - Simplify

Much of what we have come to learn has been passed down from coach to coach, which we readily accept. Most of the time we do not even know why we are doing a certain exercise but because others are doing it so do we. This usually happens for the sake of variety, which is another myth about our bodies. Our bodies do not need variety - they need stimulus.

So much exercise is wasted effort with no real benefit except for some sweat due to "getting your heart rate up." Your body is producing a reactive response rather than an adaptive response. One makes you feel out of breath, sweaty, and exhausted. The other hurts.

If the reason for adding 'variety' to your training is for motivational purposes then this is the wrong approach to take. If you need to be motivated to exercise then your outlook on exercise needs to change.

Put more effort into a few basic exercises instead of having minimal effort spread across many exercises.

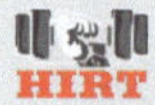

Work each set to positive failure - Intensity

As mentioned before your body does not recognize time as such. It does not have a clock inside of it that says you have worked for an hour so it is time to burn fat and build muscle. What it does recognize is intensity of effort. There are many levels and formulas to measure intensity.

You may have seen intensity described as a % of your 1RM, a % of your maximum heart rate, or even reps in reserve during a set. These are all great ways to measure and quantify your progress but sometimes they cannot give a clear indication of true intensity.

If you are doing three sets of 10 repetitions at 80% of your 1RM but are able to complete a few more reps past this, have you really worked at 80% intensity?

If your friend did the same exact workout with the same load of 80% of a 1RM but could not complete the 10th rep has he/she worked at 80% intensity?

There are too many variables to consider with the theory that intensity is measured as a % of 1RM. You may have had a higher tolerance for exercise-induced pain or you may have a higher proportion of slow twitch muscle fibers, which causes you to fatigue slower.

The levers of your limbs may be different. The speed at which you lifted the weight may have been different. This is why intensity is hard to measure on a broad scale and perhaps performing a set to Momentary Muscular Failure may give you a better indication of your true strength potential.

Be honest with your efforts & yourself - Focus

As with most successful achievements in life, you need to be focused. There is no compromise. When you study for an exam or have deadlines at work, you put great effort and concentration to get good results. The same approach needs to be taken with exercise. You need to focus on every single rep, set, and exercise you are doing.

You need to be honest with yourself and ask the tough questions - Did I work to positive failure? Could I have completed another rep with good form? Was the weight challenging enough? Was I in control of the movement or did I use momentum?

You need to be in your zone and have no distractions. No looking at the TV, changing the music channel, or planning the weekend with a friend.

If you train with a friend then make sure you are both on the same page of discipline.

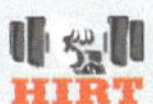

Do not rush the set - Rep Range

Let me be clear. Strength can be developed at any speed and with various ranges. There are so many methods of periodization, intensity percentage, and equipment modalities. What you are looking for is the most efficient and least complicated way to get strong in the safest way possible.

There are no compromises to safety unless you are sport requires you to specifically handle the weight a certain way i.e. CrossFit, Strongman, Powerlifting, and Olympic lifting.

We know that there must be a certain volume of mechanical work to cause significant inroad (micro-trauma) between your muscle fibers. We also know that the lower body and bigger muscle groups require a little more volume than the upper body musculature.

The lower body can accommodate a repetition range of 12 to 15 reps (sometimes up to 20 depending on the sequence) while the upper body requires a little less of about 8 to 12 (sometimes up to 15 depending on the sequence).

Keep in mind that you do not need to stop the set at that number if you still have one or two more reps left in you. This is just an indication that you are stronger and will need to increase the weight on your next session. If you cannot reach the lower end of the repetition range then the weight is too heavy and you need to go lighter.

Remember, you still need a certain volume of mechanical work and metabolic stress to stimulate an adaptive response.

Control the weight - Reduce Momentum (Rep Speed)

This is perhaps one of the most controversial topics in lifting weights - how fast should you be lifting the weight. One of the biggest myths in weight training is that if you move the weight fast you will become fast. This is a very broad statement because the question must be asked - what are you trying to get fast for?

Doing squats fast will not make you a fast sprinter. Working on your sprinting technique, take off skill, stride efficiency, and foot placement combined with your genetic ability will make you a fast sprinter.

If you make your legs (and other muscles involved in the movement) as strong as possible you have all the ingredients of becoming as fast as your ability allows you to.

Strength can be developed at any speed so why not choose the safest option, which reduces the risk of injury and ensures you recruit every available muscle fibers involved in the movement?

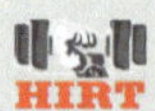

The safest way to lift weights is slow, smooth, and with complete control of the resistance. This means not allowing the weight to be airborne at any stage of the movement.

Why? Because with acceleration and increased momentum you expose your body (joints, tendons, ligaments, muscles) to a force it is not capable of withstanding. The force was produced by the acceleration of the mass NOT by the contraction of the muscles.

Think of muscular contraction as two pieces of Velcro coming together. If you bring them together slowly and with complete control, you can make sure that the little attachments (cross-bridges) interlock together and are securely attached. If you try to close a Velcro strap too fast, you do not get all the tiny attachments interlocking and the Velcro connection is not as strong.

Your muscles work the same way. As they encounter a resistance and have to produce a force to lift, hold, or lower that resistance tiny cross-bridges form between the actin and myosin filaments. The slower the contraction (less momentum & more time under tension) the more cross-bridges form resulting in the sequential recruitment of more muscle fibers. The result is a greater inroad (micro-trauma) of the muscle fibers & cross-bridges.

The argument here may be that if you work your muscles faster, you recruit the fast twitch muscle fibers but if you work your muscles slow you recruit the slow twitch muscle fibers. Slow and fast twitch has nothing to do with the speed at which they are recruited, but rather, the rate at which they fatigue.

Your slow twitch muscles are slow to fatigue and quick to recover while your fast twitch fibers are fast to fatigue and slow to recover. The only way to get to your fast twitch fibers is by going through the sequential order of slow to fast, which occurs as fatigue sets in and the load becomes more challenging.

So what is the optimal speed for repetitions? Anything above two seconds is a good starting point. When starting out a 2/2 cadence is usually effective but as you become stronger and your body begins to adapt you need to look for a greater stimulus. A 3/3 cadence is quite common or even a 4/4. Some programs will require a 5-second lift and a 5-second lower or perhaps a 2-second lift and a 4-second lower.

The main thing to remember is that you can maintain complete control through the whole range of motion and you are able to change direction of the movement with no bouncing, heaving, or jerking of the weight.

You want your muscles to be engaged throughout the whole repetition eliminating as much momentum as possible.

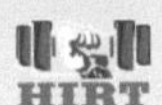

Work the whole body - 1 System

Your body operates as a complete system so it would make sense to exercise it that way. The objective here is to recover your body on rest days and not just certain body parts. Systemic recovery is just as important as localized recovery of the worked body parts.

You do not want to be spending every day at the gym working different body parts when it is not necessary. Your muscles do not require that much work.

Even though you work your legs, there is an indirect effect on your upper body. This means that when you squat with your legs you squat with your whole body. When you curl with your arms, you curl with your whole body.

Obviously the smaller the muscle group the less indirect effect on neighboring muscles which is why it's important to work from big to small as one system and then recover as one system.

By doing this, you will also maximize the potential for intensity, leading to a greater stimulus for the release of growth hormones and testosterone.

The greater the stress the greater the chance for adaption providing adequate time is given for recovery.

Look for the stimulus - Top Ups, Drop Sets, Forced Reps

As you progress through your training, there will come a point where your strength will surpass the capability of the equipment you are using. As your legs get stronger in the squat, you may not be able to load more weight on your back. Another example would be the Lat pulldown machine. Your grip and arms will give out before your Lats do.

This is where you need to look for alternative ways to reach positive muscular failure so as not to stall your progression. You want to be producing an adaptive response not a reactive response from the exercise. There are a number of ways to do this.

Drop Sets is where you progress through the set but each time you hit positive failure you immediately reduce the weight by a small margin and continue on (no rest). You should only do this once or twice in the working set. Remember the range that you are working in for upper and lower body.

Top Up is where you have another exercise ready for the same body part where you can 'top up' two or three more reps to reach muscular failure. Again do not do this for every exercise but perhaps for one or two where you feel you are lagging in development or have an obvious weakness.

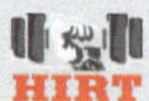

Forced Reps is simply having a good spotter to help you through the last one or two reps (especially at the sticking points). The spotter will usually assist you in the concentric phase of the lift but allow you to do it on your own on the eccentric phase of the lift (still keeping an eye on you and being ready should the need arise).

Pre-exhaust (a method devised by Arthur Jones) is where you fatigue through an isolation exercise the intended muscle and then use a compound movement for further stimulus or vice-versa (post-exhaust).

This is extremely beneficial if you have a weakness in an area of your body that limits you from stimulating a larger muscle because the smaller muscle fatigues before it. An example of this would be the squat. Your back will always be the limiting factor.

Your legs are capable of lifting much more than what your back can withstand. To combat this problem you may perform leg press or leg extensions and then move onto the squat.

You will find that your legs are already fatigued from this pre-exhaustion exercise and you will not need to lift as much on the squat. Your legs will fatigue before your back does or even at the same time.

08. *Minimize Rest - Maximize Intensity*

The bottom line is too much time is spent at the gym in between sets and exercises. Your aim is to maximize intensity to capitalize on the anabolic (growth) process, which is present when your body is put under immense stress, especially in the absence of oxygen (anaerobic metabolism).

Since we are trying to recruit the higher threshold muscle fibers we need to make sure we are not resting too long where our slow twitch fibers recover and continue to partake in the movement (remember the slow twitch are slow to fatigue but quicker to recover).

Initially when people begin to exercise, they will see immediate gains in strength, which is usually due to an increase in neuromuscular efficiency and the recruitment of the slow twitch fibers. After a while, progress stalls because people are not tapping into their fast twitch fibers to produce bigger results.

After performing a set, you usually regain 50% of your strength within 5 seconds but regaining 100% of your strength takes a few minutes. You want to minimize this time enough so that you keep recruiting the fast twitch fibers but not too short that you are completely gassed to even attempt the next exercise. Less than 60 seconds is usually the best guideline but take more time if you need to.

With a shorter amount of rest, you have built in the 'cardio' component into your workout meaning you are placing an increased demand on your cardiorespitory system.

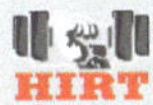

09. *Keep accurate record - Tracking progress*

How do you know where you are going if you do not know where you are starting from? To know how you are progressing you need accurate record keeping. This will ensure you are always heading in the right direction while giving you an indication if you have stalled in your development.

This is usually a sign that you need to enhance your stimulus or you just need a break from training. Yes, it is ok to take a break from training for a few weeks. If you are still progressing and not burnt, keep going.

---

10. *Recovery*

I do not like using the word 'overtraining'. Instead, I like to think of it as 'under recovered'. Once we begin to understand that your body does not grow in the gym, we will see less people burning out from exercise.

Every time you exercise, your body thinks you are trying to harm it. It calls upon its recovery reserves to treat the 'injured' area and give it a little more (over compensation) for the next time this perceived 'threat' attacks again.

It is not just your muscles that are 'attacked' but your Central Nervous System is under 'threat'. This is called a systemic inflammatory response. Your muscles produce a local inflammatory response.

You will notice that when you have been training for a while and you have not had enough rest it is actually easier to fall sick because your immune system is weaker.

Again, every time you exercise your body feels like it is being attacked so your immune system becomes inflamed to protect itself. Unfortunately, this makes you more susceptible to illness.

Further to this, you begin to place an enormous amount of stress on your Central Nervous System, which is the command center between your brain and your muscles (via the spinal cord).

That unmotivated feeling you get or the mental exhaustion you are feeling is usually a result of this. The best guide for recovery is having a day off in between sessions and at least two days off once in the week.

An example would be training Monday, Wednesday, Friday, and then have Saturday, Sunday off. By doing this, you are giving your body enough time to enhance the recovery and growth process (everything else being equal i.e nutrition, sleep, etc).

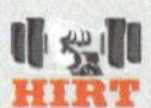

PART TWO:
PREPPING AND MOBILITY

Before we start any training regime, it is always advisable to commence with what we call prepping & mobility exercises. Not only will this provide you with the correct physical preparation but it allows you to set the right mental environment for your training i.e. focus, concentration, and visualization of what is about to occur.

Prepping is more than just 'warming up'. You want to start setting up the neurological pathways to your muscles which are about to produce force & create movements. Further to this, you will raise the temperature of your muscles which helps reduce friction during movements especially around your joints and connective tissues.

You do not need to do a lot of these at the start, as you do not want to compromise your strength for the main part of the session. A few reps of each with good technique will suffice.

01. *Hollow Rocky*

This abdominal exercise has many uses including a neural strength platform to prep yourself before heavy lifting. As the name suggests you are creating a hollow platform while lying on your back and rocking back and forth without losing the engagement of the minor muscles of the hips and torso.

- Lie on the ground with lower back touching the surface

- Legs must be straight and tight together with toes pointed away from you

- Arms straight behind you keeping your biceps close to your ears

- Start rocking back and forth without allowing your body shape to break at any point

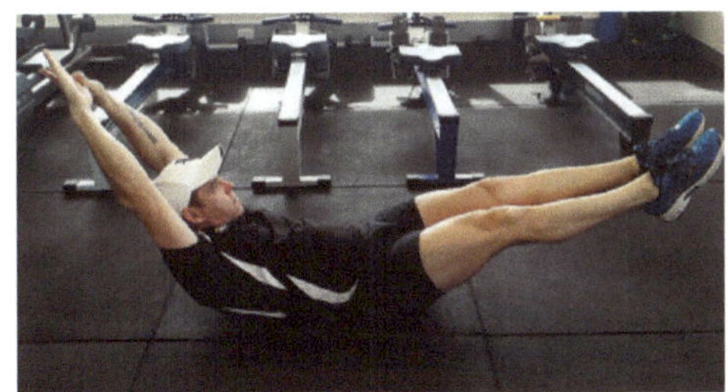

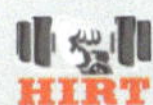

02. **Knees to Elbows**

Knees to elbows is a hanging strength exercise that incorporates strength from your core center of gravity (hips/torso) to your shoulders. It is commonly used for Pull Ups and toes to bar progressions.

- Start by hanging with your arms straight off a chin up bar
- Do not have your arms out too wide. Straight above you is sufficient
- Without swinging or rocking bring your knees towards your elbows
- Do not bend or use your arms but try to engage your as much of your torso to lift your knees
- Lower them back down slowly

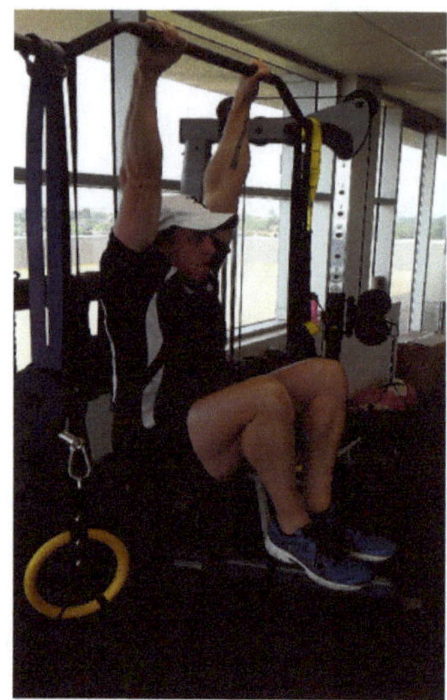

03. **Side Plank**

The side plank is a basic isometric exercise that is incorporated into a strength program to facilitate core strength as well as spinal and shoulder stability. It is the basic movement of holding your body on its side where your center of gravity (core) is forced to work as it tries to hold the bulk of the load.

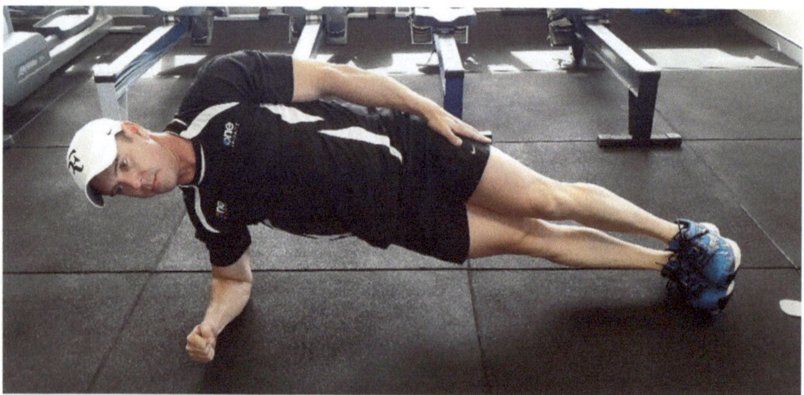

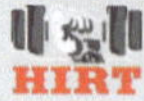

04. *Shoulder Touches*

The shoulder touch exercise is another core and shoulder strength exercise that utilizes a large amount of stability and accuracy. Starting in a push up position with your hands directly under your shoulders and in line with your chest try touching your opposite shoulder or even the same side.

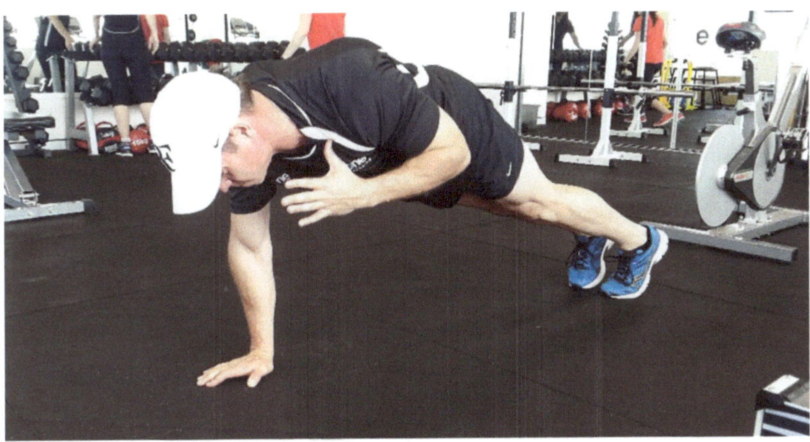

05. *Bottom of Squat Balance*

The bottom of squat balance exercise is a very useful tool in prepping your squat and increasing the ability to drive out of a full squat with the appropriate posterior chain tension. You can begin by standing in front of a pole or holding a broomstick and lowering yourself into a full squat position.

·Keep your heels/feet flat on the ground
·Raise your chest up so it's facing the pole/stick
  • Slight anterior pelvic tilt as you lower your body into the squat

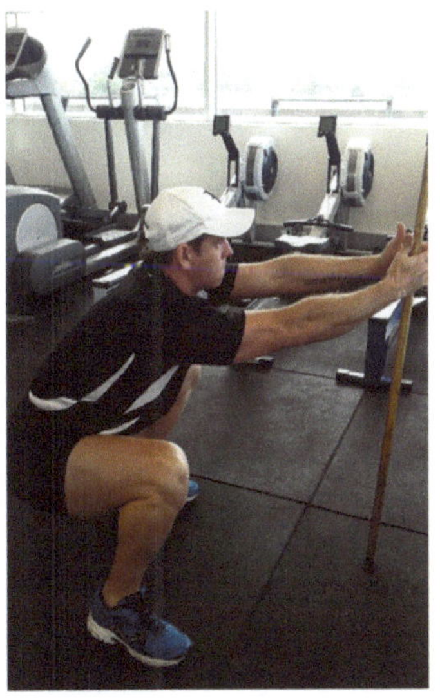

06. *Shoulder Dislocations*

The shoulder has the most range out of all the joints in the body but it comes at a price. It sacrifices stability. This being the case it's important you work on improving the strength of all the muscles surrounding the shoulder joint using a full range of motion during exercises.

Before you do this, you want to make sure you work on your mobility and range which can be done by some simple rotational work around the joint.

- Hold a broomstick in front of you with your arms straight and wide
- Without bending at the elbows bring the stick over your head rotating around the shoulder so the stick is now behind you
- Bring it back over without hitching your shoulders up and bending your arms
- As you improve your mobility and range of movement you will be able to bring your hands in closer along the stick

---

07. *Inch Worms/Caterpillar Crawls*

Sometimes used as a 'core' exercise we prefer to use the inchworms as a mobility warm up. This is a great movement, which allows you to actively stretch out some tight spots around your hips, shoulders, and ankles. It requires you to get close to the ground and engage multiple muscle groups around multiple joints.

- Stand with your feet close together. Keeping your legs straight, stretch down and put your hands on the floor directly in front of you. This will be your starting position
- Begin by walking your hands forward slowly, alternating your left and your right. As you do so, bend only at the hip, keeping your legs straight
- Keep going until your body is parallel to the ground in a pushup position
- Now, keep your hands in place and slowly take short steps with your feet, moving only a few inches at a time
- Continue walking until your feet are by hour hands, keeping your legs straight as you do so
- If you have really tight hips & hamstrings then start by bending your knees slightly

PART THREE:
THE EXERCISES

08. *Pull Up*

This well known, basic bodyweight exercise, in its many forms, is a great way of increasing your upper body and core strength. To be able to lift your total body mass through the pulling actions of your arms shows great strength of the upper body.

To be able to engage the major muscles of your torso as well as the smaller surrounding muscles to execute a Pull Up requires skill as much as strength. There is a progression system for the Pull Ups, which will help you achieve this movement.

- Hollow Rock
- Hold the bar as if you're going to break it in half
- Lift Chest
- Point Toes
- Squeeze Lats
- Pull Slowly

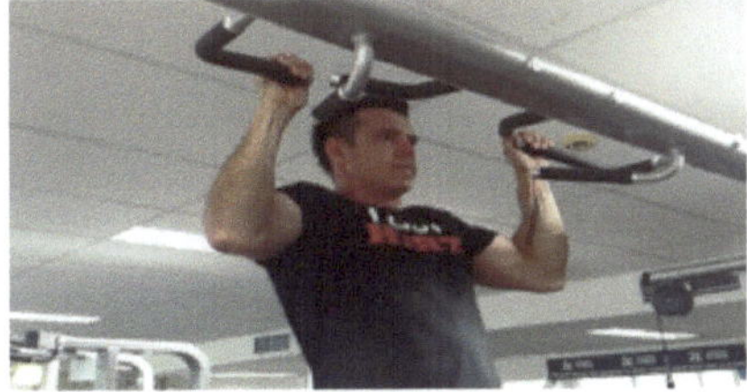

Now put it into action with these progression steps;

- Hang from top and bottom
- Jumping Hang
- Negative Hanging
- Positive Hanging
- Negative Reps

09. *Chin Up*

The Chin Up should follow the same progression as the Pull Up with the only difference being that you have a reverse grip (palms facing up). You will tend to engage your biceps more in this movement, which are the gateway to the muscles in your back. You may find it easier to start with the Chin Up before the Pull Up.

10. *Ring/TRX Row*

Simple suspension pulling exercises like the ring row and TRX row are great exercises to increase upper body strength by focusing on the back, shoulders, forearms and biceps. They also present a great progression to pull ups.

This is necessary exercise in your training. Think of it like the reverse of a bent over row but this time you are using your body as a loaded barbell without the pressure of fatigue on your lower back.

11. *Toes to Bar*

Just like the Knees to elbow exercise, toes to bar is an advanced bodyweight tool that incorporates your full body by hanging from a bar and slowly pulling your legs up to touch your toes to your hands. Think about what you're actually doing here;

You are using the lower part of your body as a resistance to load the upper body. The only way to do this effectively is by being able to hang off something (by your arms) so you're completely isolating the muscles in your back and arms to do all the work without the support of your legs.

12. *Push Ups*

This is probably the most common exercise ever utilized. It looks great in photos and always presents the 'struggle' of the participant. A lot of this probably has to do with the way the Push Up is portrayed in all those army movies. However, the Push Up is so much more than that.

It is an exercise that you actually have a conversation with. It is just you and the ground looking at each other. I see it as a game of 'Chicken' with gravity. Who will give up first? The basic Push Up is just a straight up and down action but where most people go wrong is thinking that it is just an arm and chest workout. The Push Up is a total body workout.

While your upper body is performing a concentric and eccentric contraction, your lower body (and lower torso) should be performing an isometric contraction. Your body should be moving up and down as flat as possible in one complete movement as if it was a table being lifted evenly off the ground.

A key point with the Push Up is making sure your arms and hands are not too far out in front of the body but rather are kept in line with your chest on the perimeter of your body (not on the outside).

13. Decline Push Up

As with most exercises you will only progress on them if you keep increasing the stimulus that they've adapted to. To do this you always need to look at ways of increasing the resistance or manipulating the repetition speed and range of motion. The Push Up is no different. You will become stronger and you will have more endurance so you need to find ways to alter the leverage to create more resistance.

As it's our upper body performing the mechanical work with concentric and eccentric contractions we need to find a way to increase the resistance they're subjected to. The simple solution is by having the legs and feet raised a little higher to tip the load towards the upper body.

This is done by placing your feet on a small step or bench. As you tip the load towards the upper portion of the torso, you will also increase the workload of the shoulders.

14. Deficit Push Ups

As with the need of increasing resistance and leverage another great way to manipulate the stimulus is by varying the depth and range of motion of a movement. While full ROM is always encouraged, it can be hard at times due to the mechanical structure of the body or the equipment you are using.

For example with the Push Up you have the ground to contend with so one way to combat this problem and get more depth is by creating more distance between you and the ground.

The best way to do this is by having handles on the ground, which you can hold onto. You can use two steps side by side or perhaps even specifically designed handlebars.

This extra distance from the ground will allow you to get more depth in your movement to stimulate the muscles further.

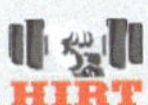

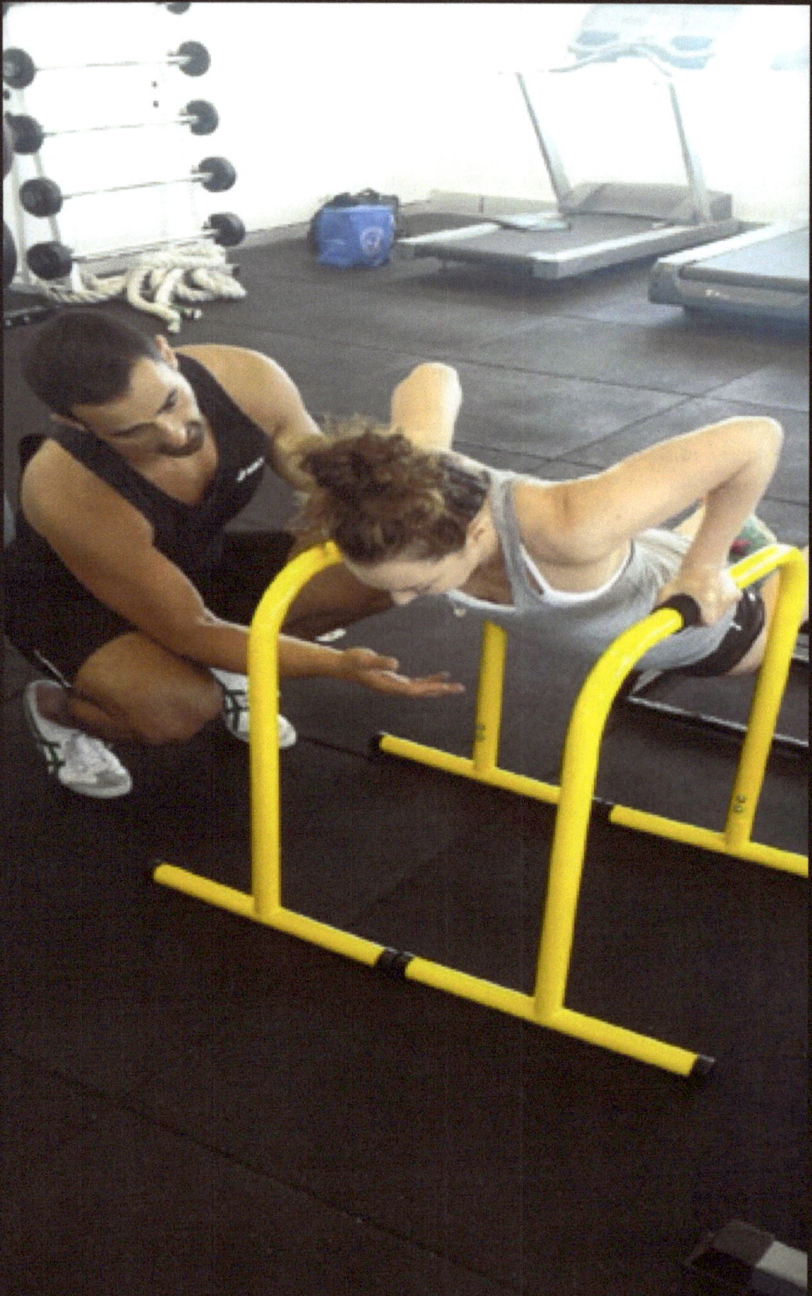

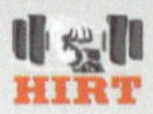

15. *Leg Extensions*

You have probably been told a hundred times not to do Leg Extensions because they are not functional or they are bad for the knees. Well I can think of many other exercises, which are bad for the knees, if done incorrectly.

While the Squats, Deadlifts, and Leg Presses are great exercises and will engage more muscular coordination and muscle fiber recruitment there is nothing wrong with isolating the Quadriceps from time to time if you find yourself lagging in development in some parts of your upper legs.

Most people when they do a Squat or Deadlift get overwhelmed by the skill of the movement that they do not properly engage all the required muscles. Further to this, they tend to place a lot of load on their lower back, which will fatigue way before their legs ever do.

A Leg Extension is a great way to show people how the muscles in the Quadriceps contract and where some of the load needs to be distributed during the bigger compound exercises.

It is also a great rehabilitation tool for increasing the load capacity of the tendons around the knee, which may have been compromised due to a knee injury or operation. Where people go wrong with the Leg Extension is they move the weight too fast and tend to bounce it at the bottom and top of the movement.

People also rest the pads too low towards their feet, which increases the torque around the knee. The pads should be resting up closer towards the shin to engage more of the quadriceps/tendons and less of the complex knee structure.

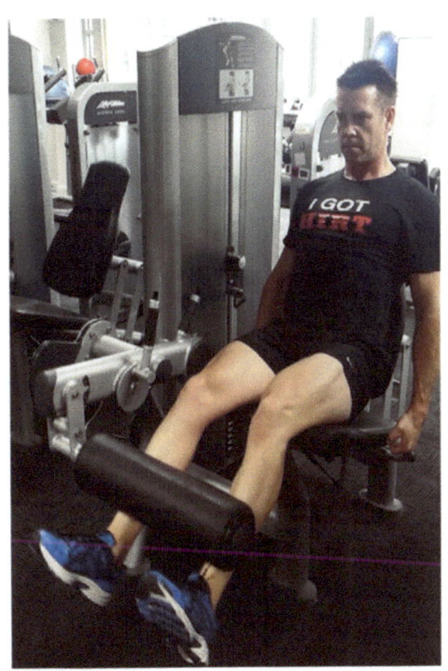

You are able to manipulate the Quadriceps muscles used in the Leg Extension by slight angle adjustments of the leg and feet positioning.

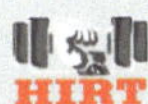

16. *Hamstring Leg Curls*

Hamstrings can be a complex muscle group to train. It is usually weaker than the Quadriceps muscle group and has a higher tendency for injury due to the in balance between the posterior thigh and anterior thigh.

This is quite common in most of the population hence why specific hamstring exercises are necessary such as Dead Lifts, Nordic Curls, and Lying Leg Curls.

While the Dead Lift is a superior exercise, it can be hard for beginners to understand what they are actually trying to do with their hamstring. Most of the time they will lead with their back and be put off the Dead Lift if they hurt themselves.

The Lying Hamstring Leg Curl allows you to isolate the part of the leg you want them to 'use' when performing a Dead Lift. Obviously, the movement pattern and skill is completely different but at least you are making them aware of where their hamstrings actually are.

The important thing to remember is not to bounce the weight up and not to allow full extension of the knee at the bottom of the movement. The pad must also be as close to the calf muscles to minimize stress around the knee joint.

This is one of our favorite exercises when we want to take a break from the Dead Lift or have stalled in our progress and requires some extra stimulation.

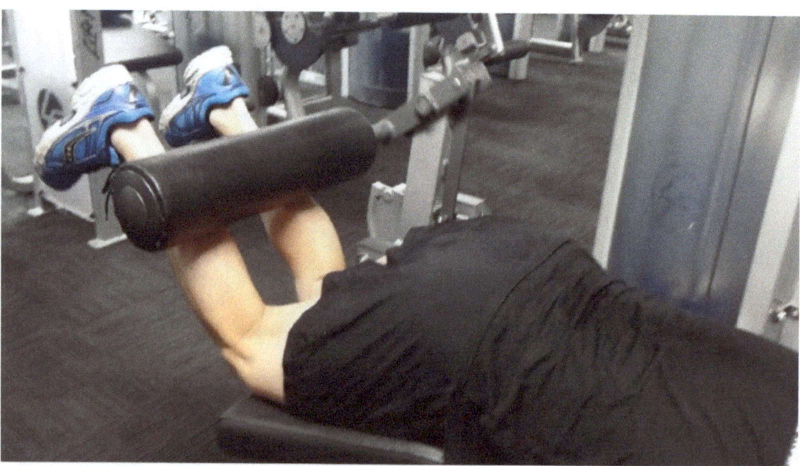

17. *Dumbbell Pull Overs*

One of the main issues when working the muscles of your upper back is that it requires your hands, forearms, and upper arms to assist with the movement. They are the gateway to the back.

Unfortunately, these are a hindrances on the development of your back because they will tend to fatigue or 'give out' before your back ever does. They can limit your ability to get a good stimulus for the Lats, Traps, & Rhomboids.

Unless you have access to a Pullover machine that takes your limbs out of the equation, there really is no other way to isolate your back. What we can do is try and replicate the movement of a Pullover machine by using a Dumbbell. By cradling the Dumbbell in the palms of both hands, you minimize the deficiency of your grip (& fingers).

By keeping your arms straight (elbows not locked) you will place more of an emphasis on using the Lats, Traps, & Delts rather than your Biceps and Triceps. These minor muscles will still be involved in the Dumbbell Pullover but they will not be as much of a limiting factor as if you were to use a rowing or pulldown movement.

A Dumbbell Pullover is great as a pre or post exhaustion exercise to your Bent Over Rows, Cable Rows, or Lat Pulldowns.

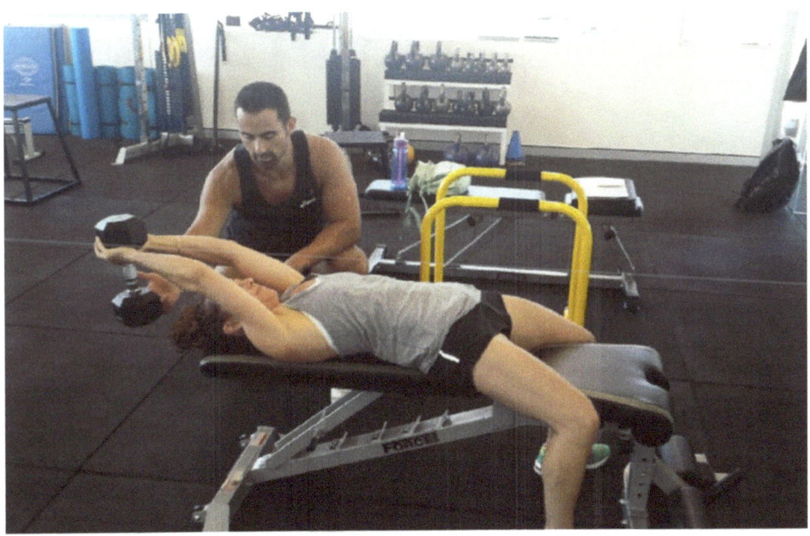

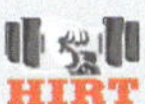

18. Pec Dec/Flys

Over the years, I have observed thousands of people train and the one thing that they all have in common when they do Bench Press is that they hit the arms & shoulders before they hit the chest. While there are many techniques involved in executing a good chest press to get deep into the pec muscles there's no escaping the fact that arms do play a major part in the movement.

One way to solve this problem is via direct resistance. That is applying direct resistance to the pectoralis muscles with an isolation exercise. You will find that you will not be able to lift as heavy because not only is it a single joint movement but you have eliminated much force generated by the arms.

The Pec Dec and Chest Flys allow you to target the intended muscle group without much support from the arms except to grip and stabilize the equipment. Once your chest muscles begin to fatigue you will not your elbows begin to bend and shift the load onto the biceps/triceps. This is a good sign whereas when you do a Bench Press your arms tend to fail before the chest and there is nowhere to shift the load because they are required in the movement.

19. Rear Deltoid Raises

Shoulders endure the most work you do with other exercises. It is involved in many movements and probably does not need as much attention as people tend to give it in the gym. There is one part of the shoulder that may need its own exercise – the rear Deltoids.

The shoulder joint has the widest range of motion, but to do so it sacrifices stability. The shoulders stability and range of motion depend heavily on its supporting structures. A small group of short muscles forms the tendon (rotator cuff) that connects the scapula to the upper arm and to the Deltoid muscle, which allows the shoulder to flex and move the arm.

If there is an overload of anterior work (chest press, shoulder press, pushups, bicep curls, etc.) then these small group of muscles that support the shoulder can be pulled forward by the much stronger anterior muscles you have been working on.

While the rear portion of your Deltoids will never be as strong as your chest muscles, it is important to develop them to their full capacity to maintain a balance between opposing muscle groups.

While back exercises will have an overlapping effect on the rear Deltoids it is still a good idea to do some isolation work to make sure you are giving them direct stimulus as there is an intricate network of muscles deep inside the shoulder and upper back region.

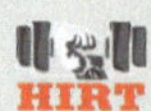

I GOT
HIRT
HAMMER STRENGTH

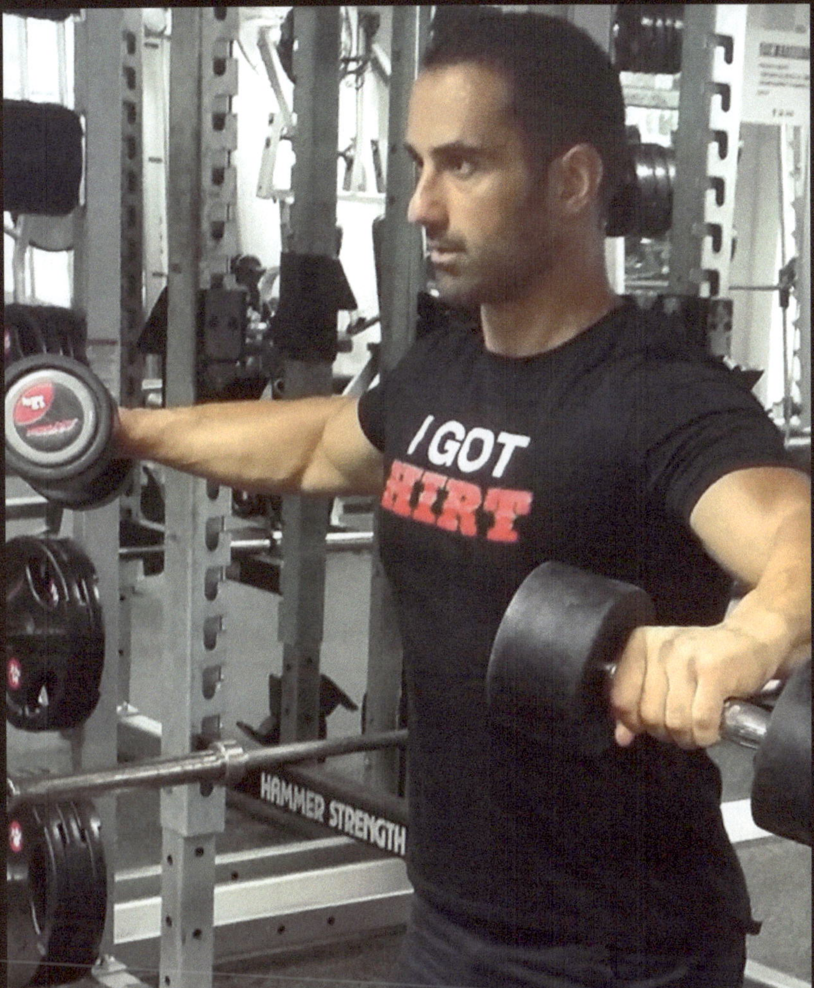

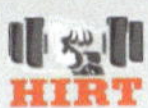

20. Triceps Extensions

Over the years, any isolated arm exercises have been deemed 'nonfunctional' for reasons that I cannot even understand, but the question I ask is how many times throughout the day do you bend your arms at the elbow? Think about how many tasks you perform which require you to use your arms.

Sure, your arms are involved in most weight lifting exercises but there is nothing wrong with isolating them from time to time. Do not forget your arms support so many other movements and are the gateway to the big lifts such as Deadlifts, Bent Over Rows, Shoulder Presses, and Bench Press.

You have to hold the bar with something and usually your hands and arms are a good start.

Tricep Extensions/Pushdowns are a great exercise to emphasize the strength in your arms as they do not necessarily 'go along for the ride' with other exercises. At times, you need to work through some weak points, which means isolating them and giving them extra attention.

21. Bicep Curls

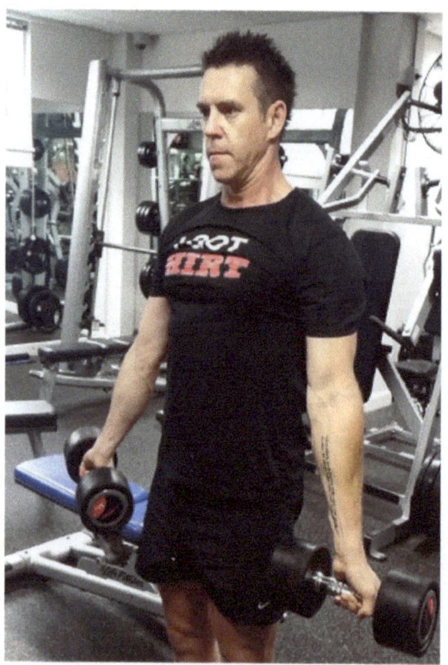

If there was ever a mistreated exercise then it has to be the bicep curl. Often ridiculed for being an ego exercise and unnecessary to do because your biceps 'get a workout' by doing the other lifts.

The biceps play an important part in shoulder stabilization due to the tendons of the long head of the biceps muscle crossing over the shoulder joint and contributing to its stability. It would make sense to increase the strength of the biceps in its complete range to help strengthen its tendons.

Increase the strength of your biceps & triceps and you will have more strength to perform the other lifts because your arms will not let you down.

22. Lat Push Downs

Along with the Dumbbell Pullover, this is probably the closest exercise to a Lat Pullover Machine (which hardly exist anymore). It will take the emphasis off your grip (to a certain extent) and force you to isolate your Lats for a greater portion of the exercise.

This exercise is best done on a cable machine with a straight bar where you can rest the palm of your hands and use your Lats to push it down. Try not to grip the bar or bend your elbows, as this will force you to use finger grip and arms to push the bar down.

Do not let your lifting ego get in the way here. You will have to start with a weight lighter than what you are usually accustomed to as you get used to the feeling of using the muscles in your back rather than the muscles in your arms and shoulders.

---

23. Dumbbell Trap Shrugs

Straight up & down. No rolling required. This is the reason why we have included this exercise in our book. To inform you that if you are going to be doing a shrugging exercise then you just need to move the weight straight up and down.

Further to this, the shrug is great for the traps even through it is called a dumbbell shoulder shrug (you have to shrug the shoulders to get to the traps).

This is one of the only exercises that hits the trapezius muscles effectively without the assistance of the arms and Lats. The initial phase of the shrug will involve the use of the deltoids, which is what makes this exercise a great all round trap and shoulder exercise.

---

24. Calf Raises

Put your hand up if you neglect these? Most of the time you hear trainers say that the calf muscles look after themselves. This is true to a degree but it is still important to include some calf strength work. Why? Because you are always on them.

They are a crucial part of your structural support when you stand. Strong calf muscles means strong ankle and knee joints. Work them.

---

25. Back Extensions

Perhaps the most limiting factor anyone will have when exercising is the weakness of his or her back. This is usually noticeable when someone is performing a squat, a deadlift, or bent over row. Their lower back muscles tend to give out before the actual prime movers.

- Lay on your stomach with your hands underneath your chin.
- Have your legs straight, feet, and hips firmly placed on the ground.
- Raise your chest slightly off the ground with a slow tempo.
- Make sure you do not bounce up but focus on using the muscles in your lower back and down the side of your spine (erectors) to raise your trunk up off the ground.

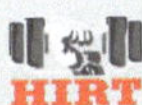

26. Leg Press (45 Degrees)

Let's face it, not everyone likes to Squat or CAN squat. There can be various reasons for this and if you come across it then you have to work around it.

You may also have someone who can squat 150kg but is reluctant to put any more weight across their neck even though the strength in their legs can handle it. Again, you need to find ways to work around it.

Think of the 45 Degree Leg Press as an upside down squat. It will take the pressure of your neck and back forcing you to isolate the muscles of the legs. When performing a Leg Press you should place your feet on the platform as if you were placing your feet on the ground for a squat.

When pushing the platform away from you your heels should push through rather than the front of your foot. Keep in mind that your knees do not want to be collapsing inwards so squeeze them out as you push the weight up.

A 45-Degree Leg Press can also be used as a 'top up' to squats. If you have a client who has fatigued on squats due to lower back fatigue then you can get them to finish their set on the Leg Press.

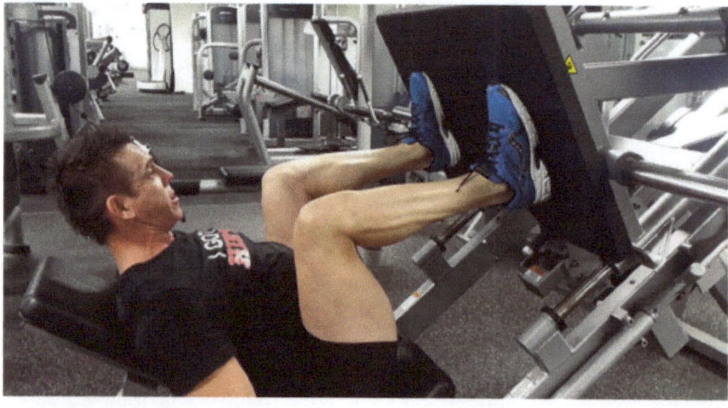

27. *Machine Seated Row*

Yes, you are sitting down and it may not be deemed 'functional' but what are we trying to do here exactly? Build strength through the muscles of the upper back. We are not concerned with balance, stability, skill specific sports conditioning, or functional everyday movements.

What limits us the most when doing a bent over row? Usually our lower back and grip strength. Yes, it is important to work on these too but occasionally you need that extra effort in your upper back without being hampered by the lower back.

I find the seated row allows me to eliminate momentum and focus on a direct path of movement for a quality stimulus. The muscles of the upper back have a lot more to give then the lower back allows it to.

- Sit upright making a 90 degree angle with your torso & lower body
- Place feet firmly on the ground
- Look straight ahead
- Eliminate swinging action
- Focus on moving the resistance with the muscles of your upper back
- Squeeze your shoulder blades into your spine
- Slowly reverse the direction

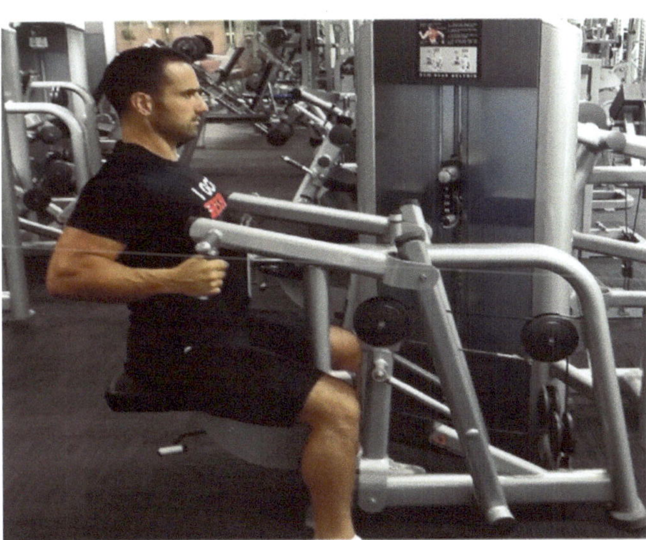

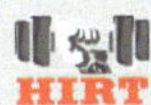

Machine Chest Press

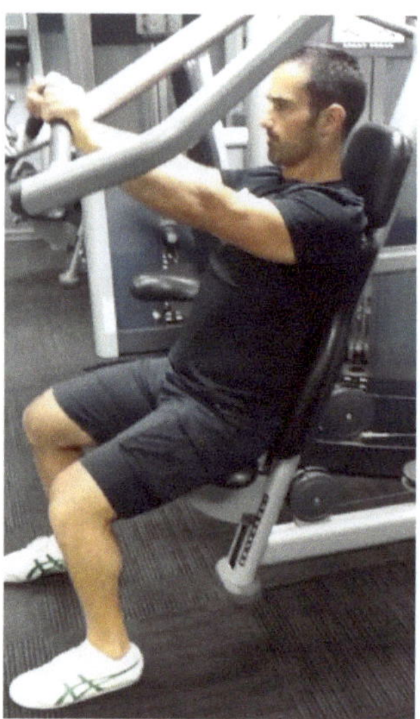

If you have access to this machine alongside a seated row machine then you are in for one epic superset sequence. The most common sequence for a HIRT session is in superset format and nothing mimics opposing muscle groups like a seated row/chest press.

The machine chest press is a great option if you are spotter-less and want to push some heavy weight through your pec muscles. The chest press machine allows you to work to positive failure without the risk of dropping the barbell on yourself.

- Sit upright
- Plant feet firmly on the ground
- Keep handles in line with your chest
- Relax the shoulders and push through your pecs
- Reverse the direction smoothly

Machine Shoulder Press

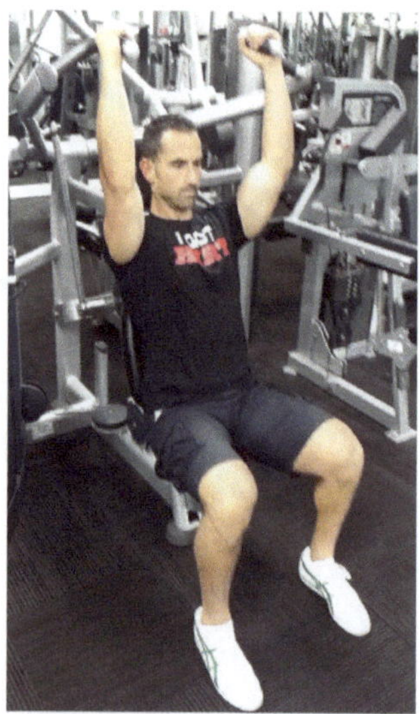

I have found that using the seated shoulder press has actually helped me press over my head better while standing because it has allowed me to work on my sticking points (the weak link in my path of movement).

30. *Narrow Grip Pull Downs*

This is one of those exercises where if you were limited to just two or three upper body exercises you would choose this as one of them. Not only does it engage multiple muscle groups it also varies the resistance through your weaker points and relies on the most dominant muscle at that point to work harder.

Beginning with Biceps, then deltoids, followed by the upper back, and finishing with triceps this is a complete upper body exercise. The key point here is not to yank the cable but control it smoothly throughout the entire range of movement.

- Use a narrow grip
- Have feet planted firmly on the ground
- Do not rock forward or backwards
- Relax the shoulders and look straight ahead

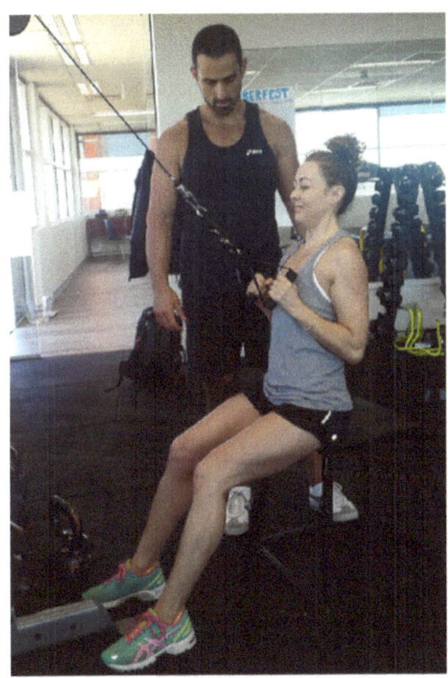

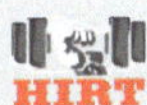

PART FIVE:
LOADED PUSH, PULLS, AND CARRIES

31. Fireman's Carry

Traditionally used as a technique in firefighting or combat, where a firefighter or soldier would carry a person over their shoulders, away from danger. This can also be used as a strength tool by lifting a large heavy object a certain distance. Instead of carrying another human being, one can use a rope or heavy sandbag of similar weight.

Important features of the carry are to keep a small gate with bent knees and brace your core muscle groups as you move.

32. Farmers Carry

A farmer's carry is a weighted carry that is traditionally used in the sport of strongman. When doing a farmer's carry, you use a piece of equipment comprised of a pair of thick metal bars with handles in the middle.

This allows you to carry the bars and gives you the ability to load weights onto each end. Conversely, you can use other equipment like Kettlebells, Sandbags and Dumbbells.

Like the firefighter's carry, a small gate with a lowered center of gravity is paramount in keeping the walk efficient. Furthermore, it is very important that shoulders are packed and retracted to stop the weight moving forward away from your body.

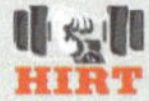

33. *Weighted Drag and Carry.*

Unlike the previous carrying exercises, the weighted drag and carry, is completed by dragging a heavy object in a backward motion. This attacks the large thigh muscles on the front of the leg as well as the big supporting muscles around your spine. This particular exercise can be executed with a heavy rope, sandbag, tyre or weighted sled.

34. *Prowler Push*

The prowler push is an exercise that uses a weighted sled called a prowler. Concentric in its nature, it is designed to strengthen and condition most of the body's muscular skeletal system via a heavy pushing movement over a certain distance (think pushing a car that has run out of fuel). There are several different positions one can use to push the prowler, from a high and upright to a low and centered position.

When used correctly, the body transverses from its anterior chain to its posterior can of muscles as you continue to step and move forward. This effect gives great stimulus to the body in aiding both a reactive and adaptive response for strength and general conditioning.

35. *Lateral Band Walks*

The lateral band walking exercise looks pretty strange (and feels strange at first), but this exercise is a great way to improve hip and knee stability as well as using neural activation of the adductors and glute medius before heavy squatting, thrusting and lifting.

The only equipment that you require is two therapy bands of different strengths. The stronger of the two bands is placed around the ankles and the second band is placed around the knees. Squat down into a 1/4 squat position as you begin to walk laterally.
An upright spine with shoulders retracted is optimal as you lead out with your knees.

36. *Duck Walk*

The Duck walk is a dynamic mobility exercise that increases the length of working tissues in the hip knee and ankle regions before squatting or thrusting. From a standing position squat deep until your glutes are almost touching the floor.

From there, begin to take small steps forward as you drive your knees out. Ensure you land each footstep upon the heel of your foot and not on your toes.

Doing 10 meter repeats is a great way of prepping your next heavy lower body lifting sequence.

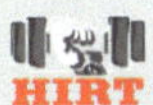

37. *Burpee.*

The Burpee is a three positional conditioning exercise that involves going from a standing position to a push up position then quickly into a full squat jump. It can be performed at different speeds to complete different objectives.

Primarily it is performed at great speed with perfect agility and accuracy to accumulate power efficiency over a given time or number of reps.

38. *Battle Rope Slams*

No doubt, you have seen this exercise on T.V, magazines, and movies, but there is a lot more to it than just waving your arms everywhere.

It is a great total body conditioning exercise forcing you to use your muscles in a chain like fashion to produce as much mechanical work as possible.

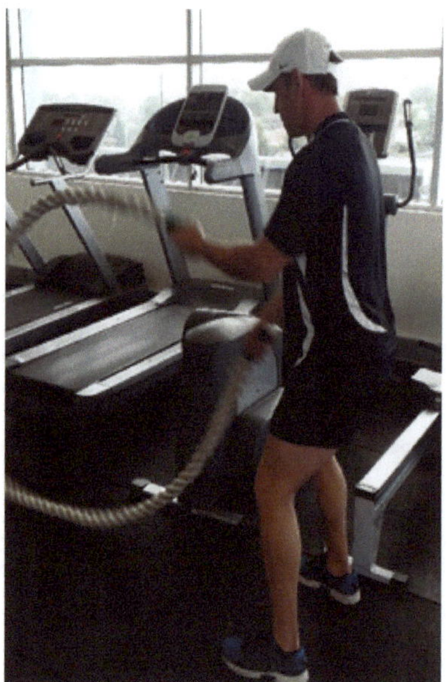

- Grabs the two ends of the rope, with either an underhand or an overhand grip
- Take about 3 to 5 steps up towards the anchor point. This puts a great deal of slack in the heavy rope. Then, in a "swing" like fashion, swings the ends of the rope up and then slams them down in order to try to force a huge wave all the way through the rope to reach the anchor point
- This requires a tremendous amount of power in both the up & down swing

There is no momentum here to take advantage of when performing the Battle Rope Slam. The user simply has to generate enough force to elicit the wave through the slack of the rope to reach the anchor point in rapid-fire succession.

39. *T-Bar Row*

The T-bar row is a back exercise that encompasses a majority of the muscles in the back and arms.

Using a T-bar machine or an unsupported T-bar plate requires an immense level of core, shoulder and elbow stability to carefully pull the weight towards your body and then slowly lower it.

This particular exercise can be used as a supplementary exercise to increase the ability to do a pull up or deadlift.

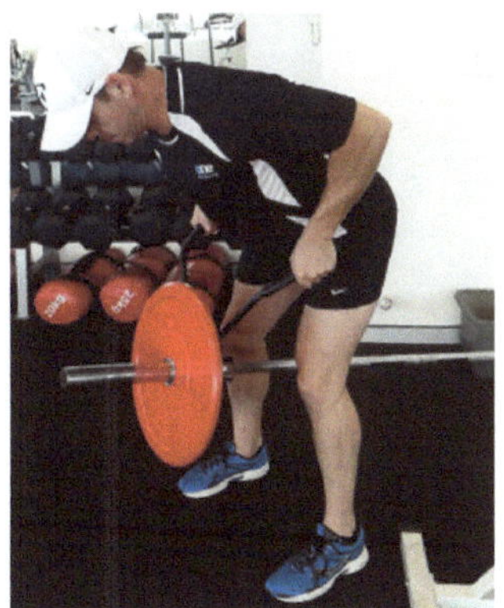

40. *Bent Over Row.*

The bent over row exercise is just like its cousin the T-bar row. However, the exercise is executed with a straight barbell and the body in a bent over 45-degree angle. A multitude of grips can be used, such as a pronated, supinated, finger lock and mixed grip.

41. *Upright Row*

In its many forms (Dumbbell, Barbell or cable) the upright row is a great pulling exercise that primarily strengthens the muscles in the shoulder region as well as upper and lower trapezius. The most common upright row, utilizes a barbell from a standing position.

Keeping your core group tight and packed, the barbell is lifted from the hang position (arms straight) until it reaches your chin and your elbows reach your ear height.

A slow and steady retraction of the bar is needed to start the next repetition. Other formats can be utilized via a seated dumbbell or standing cable position.

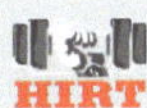
HIRT

42. Lunges.

The lunge is one of the body's most primary movements and can be used in an array of different patterns. The basic bodyweight lunge starts from a standing position, then taking a step forward place the heel on the ground at hip with and full gate.

Bend the knee and track it over your toe as your back knee bends to accommodate your weight and forward movement. Ensure your knee bends at 90 degrees before bringing yourself backward to a standing position.

---

43. Static Split

From a split and stationary stance lower your bodyweight and back knee towards the ground as you remain in a front flat foot position. To gain extra leverage you are able to raise your back foot onto a bench but ensure that the drive up is from the heel on the ground NOT the leg that is rested on the bench.

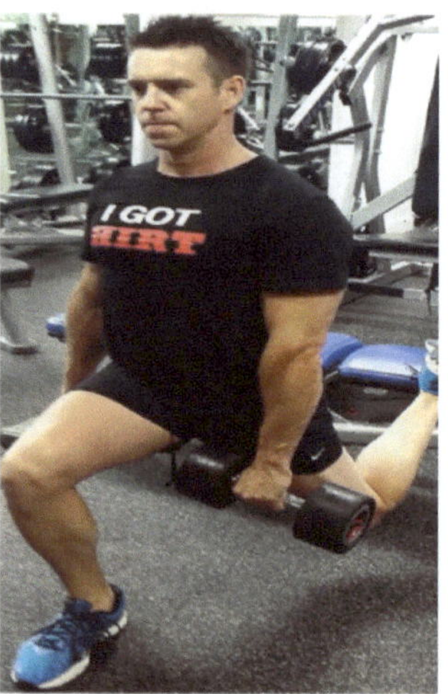

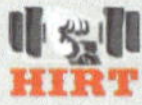

44. *Dynamic.*

The dynamic lunge or walking lunge, as it is known, can be used in many ways. One is to strengthen primary leg and core muscles and two, to facilitate dynamic mobility and movement patterns for loaded traveling exercises (sprinting, running, and carrying exercises)

45. *Back Lunge*

This lunge gets its name not via the movement but from the position that one would rest a barbell (on the back of their shoulders) Not to confuse you, but this movement can also be used in a backward, a step forward, a stationary position and a walking movement.

46. *Front Lunge*

Just like its twin, the back lunge, the front lunge is named by the position of the barbell in relation to the shoulders. In this type of lunge, the barbell is carried upon the front of the shoulders.

47. *Overhead Lunge*

The overhead lunge is an advanced lunging exercise that requires a tremendous amount of core, shoulder and hip stability.

Placing a barbell, dumbbells or any given fixed weight above the head, slowly lunge forward, backward or walk steadily over a given distance.

Prescription of this exercise is largely for advanced lifters who have no shoulder or hip impingements.

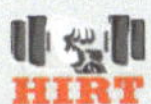

48. *Wall Ball*

The Wall Ball is a strength and conditioning exercise that involves a great deal of strength, stamina and accuracy. You start from a standing position whilst holding a weighted medicine ball. Then squat down past or equal to 90 degrees the accelerate up out of the squat and throw the ball to a target (Preferably 8ft-10ft above the ground). When the ball hits the target, wait till it falls back down into your hands then repeat.

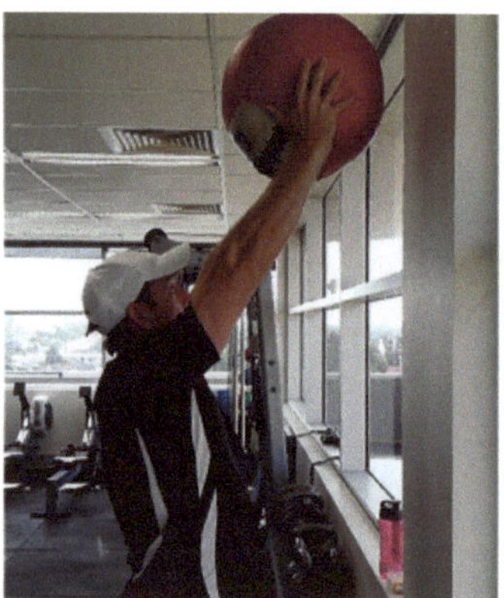
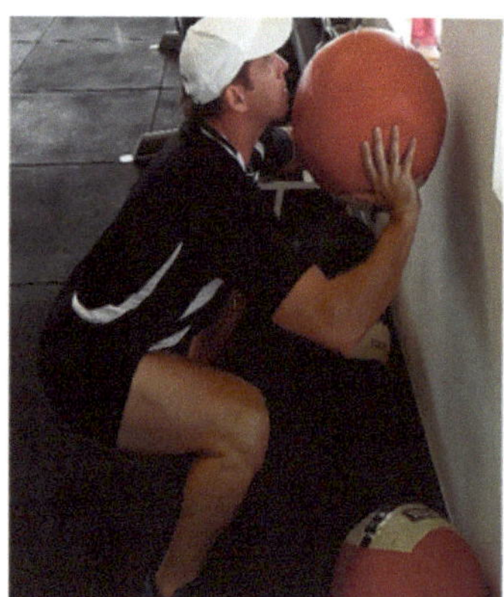

49. *Stiff Leg Dumbbell Deadlift*

While the conventional deadlift is a staple exercise in most training programs it has a younger brother that tends to get neglected – the stiff leg version. Why? Hamstrings and only hamstrings. Obviously there are other muscles involved such as glutes and erectors but this version allows you to deeply attack the muscles of the hamstring which may not receive the same treatment during a conventional deadlift.

The use of dumbbells is purely optional but we like to vary the use of barbells and dumbbells between 'family' exercises.

- Grip dumbbells using an overhand grip (palms facing down)
- Stand with your torso straight and your legs spaced using a shoulder width or narrower stance. The knees should be slightly bent. This is your starting position.
- Keeping the knees stationary, lower the dumbbells to over the top of your feet by bending at the hips while keeping your back straight. Keep moving forward as if you were going to pick something from the floor until you feel a stretch on the hamstrings.
- Start bringing your torso up straight again by extending your hips until you are back at the starting position.

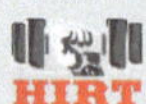

Hip Thrust

An exercise that perhaps needs to be credited to 'The Glute Guy' Brett Contreras who has brought this movement into mainstream training. If there ever was an isolation exercise for the Glutes then this is it (although there is multi joint movement through hip & knee).

While the Squats, Deadlifts, and Leg Presses are all great exercises to target the legs the Hip Thrust allows you to get deep into your Glutes without much assistance from other muscles as what tends to happen with various leg exercises.

- To perform the exercise, all you need is a low bench and a barbell
- The bar should go directly on your upper thigh, directly below your crotch.
- The pressure can greatly increase when you start lifting heavier weights so using a pad or towel helps relieve the pressure
- Once you have the bar in your lap, the next thing to do is get set up for your first repetition. I find it most comfortable to place the edge of the bench pad across the middle part of the back—right below the shoulder blades
- When you lift heavier weights, you need to use your elbows to raise your body to set up the lift
- Your feet should be directly under your knees, so when you fully extend into the lift, your knees make a 90-degree angle with the ground
- Your neck should always remain neutral
- It's important to engage your glutes throughout the lift
- The lift should be executed smoothly with the glutes lifting the majority of the weight

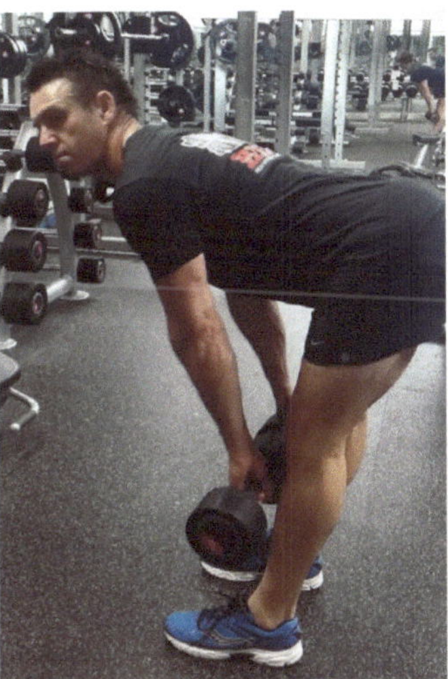

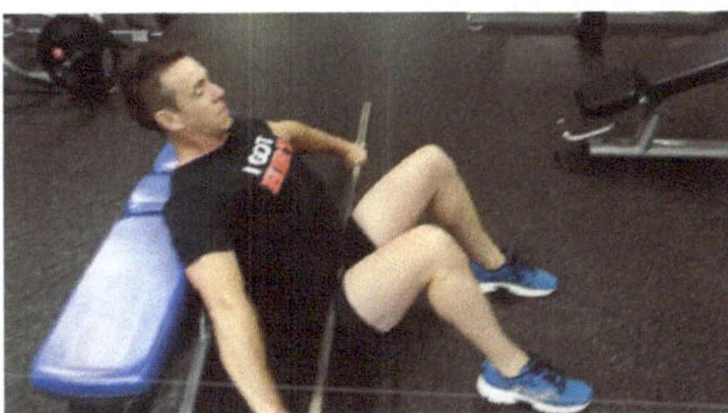

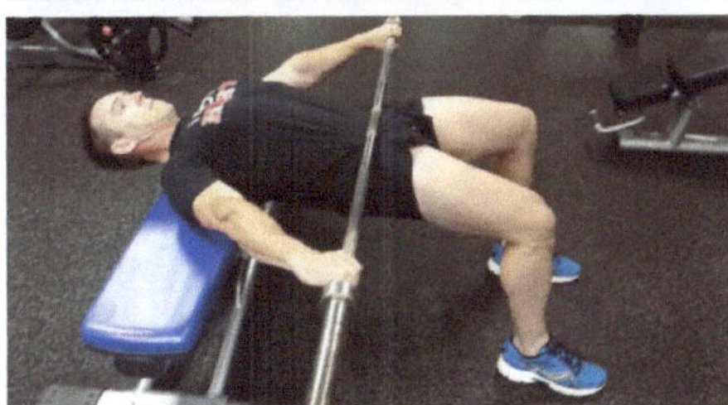

51. *Parallel Bar Triceps Dips*

Remember the statement I made about the narrow grip pulldown? If you could only choose a few upper body exercises which ones would you pick? Well this is another one of those.

The Parallel Bar Triceps Dips is an ideal upper body exercise that allows you to get deep into a range of muscle groups from the chest, shoulders, upper arms, and upper back. The key here is not to bounce up out of the bottom of the movement but to engage every muscle involved in the exercise.

The mistake most people make is thinking that this is only a Triceps exercise but done properly it is one of the most effective ways to get that extra stimulus through your chest when you fail on the bench press or chest press. It can be used as a pre exhaustion exercise or in an agonist superset sequence.

Make sure your elbows are close to your waist and you have a slight tilt forward when lowering your body into the drip. Relax the shoulders and pull your scapula into your spine as you set up for the movement.

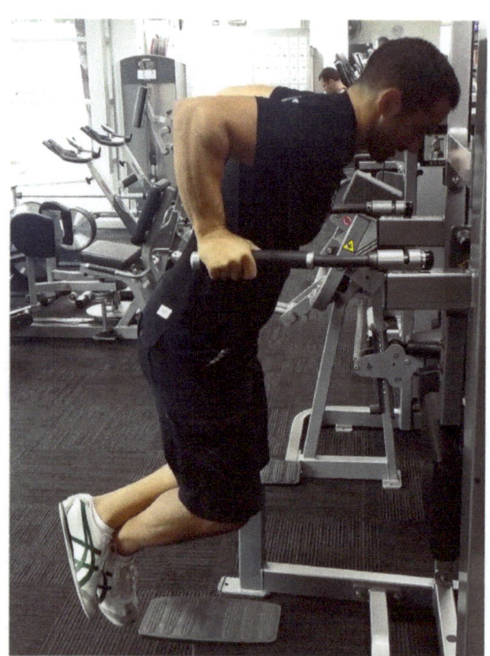

52. *Your Exercise.*

No this is not an error. We have saved exercise number 52 for the one that works for you. Through your experience, observation, and own research you may have found ways to do things which are not mainstream or considered 'functional'.

No one will know your body or the body of your clients like you so you need to take confidence in your own ability and know that you are doing something right – if it's working.

There is something that Arthur Jones (founder of Nautilus Training Equipment) used to teach and that was 'self-evident truth'. He said there are some things we do not know why or how they work but we just know they work, and when to apply it.

Intuitively he knew what was beneficial and what was outright dangerous. Our industry is filled with much negativity and criticism as it seems everyone is an expert in something and if you do not do it their way you are doing it wrong.

We want you to ignore this narrow-minded way of thinking and continue to research your methods and develop your knowledge. You will feel like you are swimming upstream at times but we implore you to keep going and believe in yourself.

> *You should understand that when participating in any exercise or exercise program, there is the possibility of physical injury. If you engage in this exercise or exercise program, you agree that you do so at your own risk, are voluntarily participating in these activities, assume all risk of injury to yourself, and agree to release and discharge HIRT and its presenters from any and all claims or causes of action, known or unknown, arising out of our courses.*